contents

hello :)

...welcome to a healthier and slimmer you...

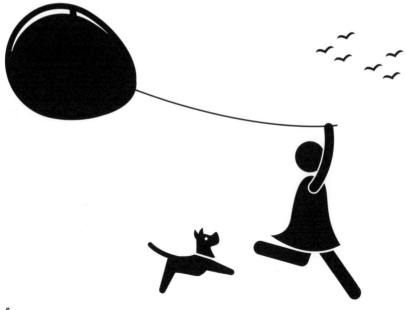

it's not fun being fat – or, to be politically correct, overweight. and i should know. once upon a time, i was seriously overweight too – in fact, i was massive.

I'm a full-time working mum. Like many in the same situation, I was time-poor and didn't make myself a priority. At my worst, I weighed over a staggering (and uncomfortable) 128kg. At 175cm tall, that made my BMI a huge 42 kg/m². In medical speak? I was morbidly obese.

To change it, I desperately needed to know what to do in order to drop weight and be healthy – fast. I was fat and getting fatter by the minute, as well as on the brink of diabetes, with hypertension (high blood pressure) and a fatty liver. My doctor was completely freaking out – and I don't blame her.

I was tired of the boring and expensive diet books that were 300 pages long but only had a couple of useful points to them. I didn't need some super-fit trainer speculating on how to lose weight from their lofty 12-pack perch – I wanted someone who *truly understood* the physical and emotional toll, someone who had lived through their own weight issues and who had also been through successful weight loss – someone who could get to the point simply and quickly. And I didn't want some of the answers – I needed all of them!

A recent report from the Australian Institute of Health and Welfare (AIHW) revealed we have one of the highest rates of obesity in the world – 25% of children and a whopping 63% of adults in Australia are overweight or obese. Interestingly, 15% *more* people are overweight in the outer regional or remote areas of Australia, compared to the cities. Scary. Australia is one of the world's fattest countries, sitting right beside the USA and the UK – it is an epidemic.

Why are more of us obese than ever before? It's obvious – we've been given the wrong advice.

According to the AIHW, 'excess weight, especially obesity, is a major risk factor for cardiovascular disease, Type 2 diabetes, some

musculoskeletal conditions and some cancers. As the level of excess weight increases, so does the risk of developing these conditions. In addition, being overweight can hamper the ability to control or manage chronic disorders.' Isn't that terrifying?

We have always been told to eat less and exercise more – for years, that has been the common-sense answer to losing weight. But... well... *what if that's wrong?* We've also been told that it's our fault we are fat – we're 'too lazy, too greedy', or we don't have the will-power, plus a barrage of other insulting stuff.

That is also a *big fat lie.*

so stop putting yourself down, and read this – i mean read it and absorb it – because this works... *fast*

Supermarkets are a minefield of sugary food and drinks – and unfortunately, the average shopper is misled again and again. How are you supposed to know what's truly healthy when every second food product is labelled 'diet', but will actually make you fatter?

There are many false beliefs about what's going to help. My method of weight loss costs nothing – it's simply a shift in how you shop and eat. And so far, I have lost 30kg (66lbs) in 30 weeks.

I know! WTF? Pause while I high-five myself!

I was uncomfortable. I was fat. I was desperate for a long-term answer – and nothing was working. So I started reading and doing research, looking at recent medical studies on losing weight, and asking the people I work with – mostly young, fit models – what they eat.

And I became my own guinea pig. When one weight-loss technique worked, I found ways to boost it. *I wanted to achieve the fastest weight loss possible without killing myself doing it.* A way of dropping the weight that

would last the long haul, as I had a lot of weight to lose.

I wanted warp-speed weight loss. When you're fat, you want the fat gone – preferably yesterday. *I wanted the fat to stay off – permanently.* This weight-loss plan had to be something I could commit to for life. A lifestyle change for the better.

Individually, these techniques are not new. But put together, just like combining hydrogen and oxygen to make water (H_2O), they're like magic. It's this *combination of techniques* that creates super-fast weight loss. And as a by-product, improved health. (Obviously, get yourself checked out by your doctor too.)

I know you have a busy life, so this book is a condensed, quick read – simple ideas that work. Big weight loss is *mostly about the food.* Exercise is important to a lesser extent – for me, it's walking and, in summer, swimming. This year in a bikini…

I follow these rules every day.

while everyone is different, here are the health benefits i gained from eating like this...

- weight loss (30kg or 66lbs... so far)
- lower risk of diabetes
- better blood pressure
- lower cholesterol
- less visceral fat (the bad fat around organs)
- less inflammation in my body
- improved liver function
- more energy
- less tired
- great mood
- glowing skin
- sharper brain
- better clothes to buy! (and i'm not invisible to shopkeepers)
- easier to run around with kids
- positive life outlook
- pride in myself
- better concentration
- people say i look 10 years younger
- looking forward to exercise
- feeling AMAZING

'great things
are not done by
impulse, but by
a series of small
things brought
together'

– vincent van gogh

here are my 'rules' that i live by every day...

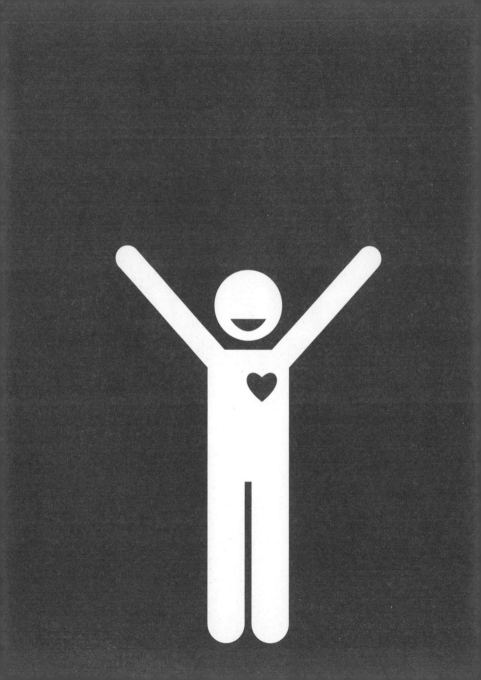

rules for the body

these rules all
contributed to my
super fast weight loss.

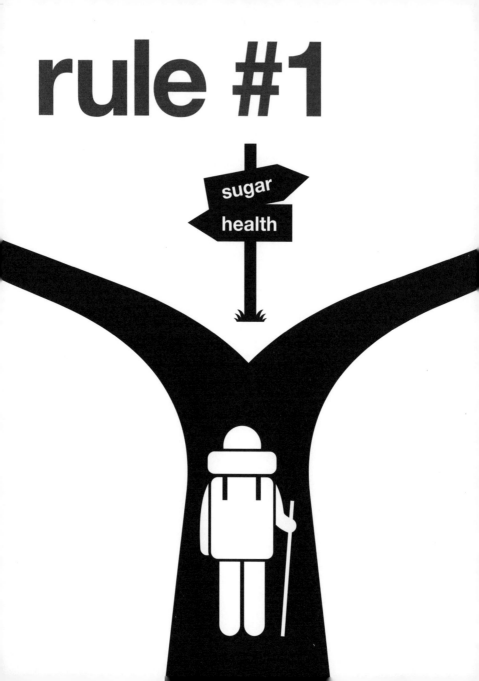

...i don't eat sugar, especially fructose...

why?

it can
make you fat.
it's that simple.

there are over 61 names for sugar, no wonder we don't even know when we're eating it.

Agave nectar, Barbados sugar, barley malt, barley malt syrup, beet sugar, brown sugar, buttered syrup, cane juice, cane juice crystals, cane sugar, caramel, carob syrup, caster sugar, coconut palm sugar, coconut sugar, confectioner's sugar, corn sweetener, corn syrup, corn syrup solids, date sugar, dehydrated cane juice, demerara sugar, dextrin, dextrose, evaporated cane juice, free-flowing brown sugars, fructose, fruit juice, fruit juice concentrate, glucose, glucose solids, golden sugar, golden syrup, grape sugar, HFCS (high-fructose corn syrup), honey, icing sugar, invert sugar, malt syrup, maltodextrin, maltol, maltose, mannose, maple syrup, molasses, muscovado, palm sugar, panocha, powdered sugar, raw sugar, refiner's syrup, rice syrup, saccharose, sorghum syrup, sucrose, sugar (granulated), sweet sorghum, syrup, treacle, turbinado sugar, yellow sugar.

Fructose is in everything. Who knew? It was a major factor to my being overweight, as I have a real sweet tooth.

Chocolate cookies would positively call my name. I could demolish a pack of Chocolate Royals in ten minutes flat. That's 93g of sugar, or about 23 teaspoons.

Sugar is not just in sweets, though. It can be found in many savoury foods, such as BBQ sauce, which can be up to 50% sugar. Isn't that an astounding fact?

Food companies call it The Bliss Point. Adding sugar to sweet *and* savoury foods to make them more palatable – and more irresistible.

Added sugars are found in approximately 75% of packaged food at the supermarket. And sometimes in things that you wouldn't expect, such as bread. The highest concentration of sugars are mostly found in these foods: sweetened beverages, baked goods, dairy desserts, lollies/candy, and wait for it... breakfast cereals. Isn't that horrifying?

I aim to stick to fewer than 3 added teaspoons of sugar a day. A teaspoon is about 4g. In general the less sugar in my diet, the faster my weight loss. This is my most important rule – I equate it to 50% of my weight loss.

this is how sugar can make you fat.

Weight gain is individual, and there are a lot of factors – like your genetics, how much exercise you do and how many calories you take in each day. But if you eat too much sugar it can be a real problem, because excess calories from sugar can be stored as fat – not great for losing weight!

A lot of people don't realise that hormones like insulin and leptin play a part in all this too. Disrupting the function of the hormones that regulate our energy levels and appetite makes us more likely to reach for that muffin or bag of lollies. Think about how easy it is to eat a heap of sweet food, and never feel full. Usually I get to the 'feel sick' stage first.

If sugar isn't used as energy by your body after eating, it will be converted into stored body fat.

It's also seriously hard to resist sugar when you're craving it. Lab studies on animals even suggest they can become addicted to it.

You will need to be strong and consistently say no to break this sugar habit but, once you have, it's an amazing difference.

Within a week or so of cutting out sugar, I found I was feeling less tired, had more energy, fewer bad moods and a more positive outlook. Added bonus: it's better for my teeth, too.

I am no longer addicted. I no longer feel the 'pull' to reach out and throw three blocks of chocolate in my trolley when shopping, then eat one on the way home. I didn't realise how hooked I was, but now it's easy to say **no**.

rule #2

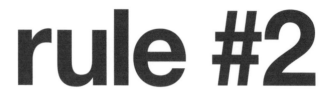

...i mostly don't eat processed foods...

unfortunately about 80% of the supermarket is processed foods.

such as:
potato chips
biscuits
chocolate bars
sauces
breakfast cereals
(most are high in
sugar)
salad dressings
canned fruit
frozen chips

and that's only a
small sample!

why?

There are heaps of processed foods in the supermarket (about 80%), which means lots of hidden added sugars, bad fats and added salt – and all these foods can make you fat. *Yes, even savoury food.*

Since the 1960s, food has been more and more processed. Think about it – pre-1960s, there wasn't much of a problem with obesity. *In fact, obesity rates have more than tripled since then.*

There also weren't many processed foods. People mostly cooked at home and ate relatively simply. Now, it's hard to go out shopping anywhere without finding food by the checkout.

shop outside the aisles – it's healthier.

remember: 1 teaspoon = 4g

When pre-packaged or processed foods were first introduced, some companies put extra sugar into their products. Sugar is cheap and compulsive, making you want to eat more and therefore buy more – it's called The Bliss Point. *Smart for business but bad for your health.*

When you eat supposed 'healthy' processed foods, you can end up consuming lots of hidden sugars, not to mention lots of synthetic chemicals – which is far from natural.

For example, an average can of baked beans has the equivalent of 5 teaspoons of sugar in it. A teaspoon is 4g.

Tomato sauce (ketchup) is full of sugar – high fructose corn syrup. Ketchup can be more than 40% sugar, plus other ingredients you wouldn't recognise. If you squirt ketchup on your hamburger, you've just added 3 teaspoons of sugar. Surprising, isn't it? Imagine sprinkling those 3 teaspoons onto your burger – that is effectively what you are doing.

The US National Health and Nutrition Examination Survey 2009–2010 says, 'Decreasing the consumption of ultra-processed foods could be an effective way of reducing the excessive intake of added sugars in the USA.' No kidding!

rule #3

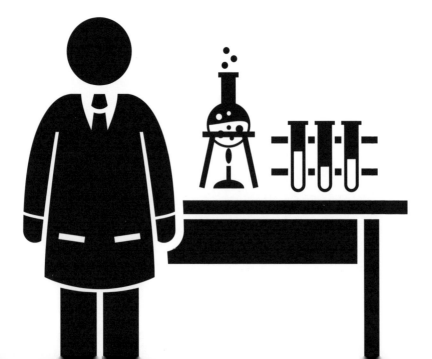

...i don't drink fizzy drinks (soda) or fruit juices, ever...

such as:
canned or bottled
soda or lemonade,
or fruit juices in
any form.

this is a really
important rule for
those who love
sweet drinks.

why?

soft drinks are chock-a-block full of sugar and they can make you fat. don't drink your way to fatness – it's easily done.

Just as an experiment, try to eat the equivalent amount of fruit that makes up a juice – say, five or six apples... You can't. It makes you full – that's the fibre filling you up.

If we were meant to juice our fruits I'm pretty sure they would have come with a straw attached – clearly they don't.

Soft drinks or soda contain about 9.5 teaspoons of sugar per can. That is about three times what I want to have in total in added sugar for the entire day!

And the sugar-free diet ones are full of chemicals such as phosphoric acid, aspartame, potassium benzonate... I don't even know what they are, let alone want to drink them.

Some people believe that there is nothing wrong with drinking a diet soda that contains zero calories. It's really up to you whether or not you are happy to consume the chemicals. For me, it is a no.

So I don't drink any of them. Except soda water.

Juices are full of fructose (sugar), without the benefit of the fibre that has been removed (the fibre is the good bit). A typical glass of apple juice has 9.8 teaspoons of sugar, which is a lot!

In short, juices have all of the sugar content (bad stuff) but none of the fibre content (good stuff). The fibre keeps your blood sugars stable and help you feel much fuller. Try not to peel your fruit, the peel contains a lot of fibre.

Which leads to the next rule...

rule #4

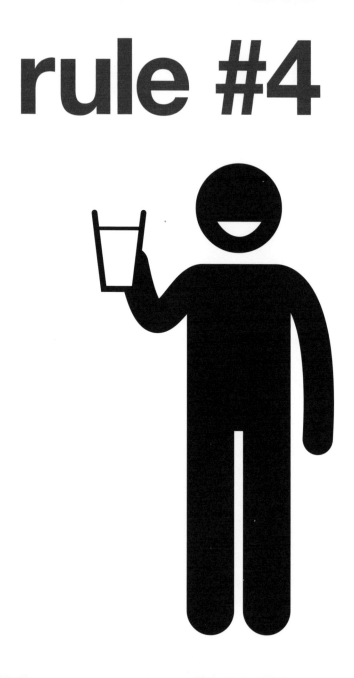

...i drink plenty of water...

why?

I drink about six to eight glasses of water a day. More in summer.

Water is essential to life. And it's essential to feeling good and dropping weight. I drink still or sparkling water and I try to aim for eight glasses a day. I find this easier to do in summer than winter. **If you feel thirsty it means you're already dehydrated**. So drink up.

I do not drink cordial or flavoured waters. I do, occasionally, put some fresh lemon into it. Try to drink water 15 minutes before eating. It makes you feel fuller and therefore eat less. I put a glass of water next to every meal to encourage me to drink it.

Drink water first thing in the morning. It sets you up for the day. Remember, water is your calorie-free friend.

Sometimes, when I'm stalking the fridge and hunting around for something, it's actually water that I want – not food. It's surprisingly easy to get mixed up with what you actually need. Sounds weird but true for me.

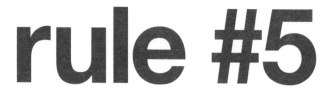

rule #5

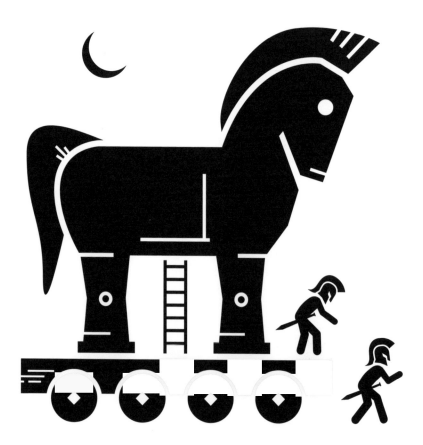

...i don't
buy diet
or low-fat
foods...

such as:
diet yoghurt
low-fat yoghurt
skim milk
low-fat milk
diet cookies
diet desserts
diet dressings

i eat:
full-fat greek yoghurt
full-fat cheese
full-fat milk
cream
sour cream
butter

why?

often diet foods contain more sugar and salt to compensate for the lack of taste from missing fats. just because they've got 'diet' in the name, it doesn't mean they're healthy!

Let's take diet yoghurt. It should really be called pudgy yoghurt – but I doubt that would sell… And as we know, it's all about what sells – unfortunately at our expense.

A popular diet yoghurt has 26g of sugar in it or 6.5 teaspoons per serve. That's more than a Mars Bar.

I try to eat as little added sugar as possible, so this is not even on the menu. No pudgy yoghurt! I usually buy full-fat Greek yoghurt or coconut yoghurt with a very low sugar content.

The same rule goes for milk, cheese – all dairy. I buy the full-fat version of everything. Natural fats fill you up and eliminate the hungry feeling.

Dairy products are a good source of calcium, protein, iodine, vitamin A, vitamin D, riboflavin, vitamin B12 and zinc.

Obviously, don't go crazy on dairy! And check the sugar and salt content. I probably consume 1 cup of milk, plus 30g of cheese a day; perhaps some sour cream and/or butter in my cooking.

There is speculation that cutting back on dairy is good for some people – this isn't the case for me, as I am not lactose-intolerant.

rule #6

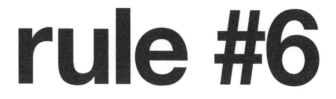
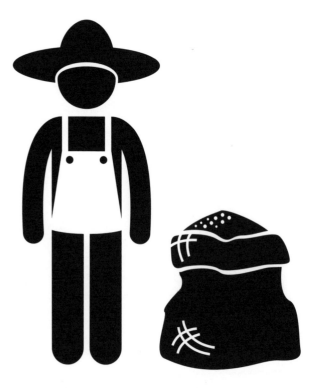

...i seriously cut back cn carbs – processed and refined... *and i mean seriously...*

why?

i do not eat white bread, pasta or white potatoes.

Breads, pastas and potatoes are all carbs that I used to love eating to excess. Athletes may need them for energy, but I am no professional athlete and I don't need that kind of energy for what I do day-to-day.

Essentially, I'm now eating lower carb. I'm certainly not saying no carb – vegetables are carbs too!

I'm saying: lower calorie, more nutritious carbs.

In general, I swap white bread, pasta and potatoes to higher fibre, more nutritious food such as vegetables, which are generally lower in calories. I want my body to use its many stored fats instead.

If you're desperate for pasta, pick up a spiraliser – it turns veggies such as zucchini (courgette) into something resembling pasta, but much healthier. They are fun to use – my daughter loves it.

Breads can be tricky. I don't know about you, but I have a love affair with bread. You need to check the label, as many have hidden sugars – or better still, bake your own (see Bern's Simple High Protein Bread Recipe on the facing page). I know, it sounds tedious – but it's actually really quick. A home-baked loaf takes me about ten minutes to make and lasts me a week.

I bake with lentil or chickpea flour, which are both higher in protein and fibre and have about one-quarter the carb content of regular flour. And they're gluten-free – if you're into that. I eat two slices of my protein bread a day and it's seriously yum and filling.

Put simply, your body requires more energy to process protein (such as fish, meat, eggs, etc). About double, in fact. It's called the thermic effect. So, think lean protein and natural fats, with a large healthy dose of vegetables and water. This will make you feel fuller longer.

Eating this way will make you less sluggish, as your blood sugars will be more balanced – I have fewer peaks and troughs throughout the day. I also don't feel bloated at all and I find that I actually have more energy for longer!

bread

Swap to a bread made with chickpea, quinoa or lentil flour – significantly lower in carbohydrates than white flour, but higher in protein, iron and fibre, and will make you feel fuller longer. Better still, bake your own. I eat no more than two slices a day.

potatoes

Swap white potatoes to sweet potatoes, which have a higher vitamin content. I would only eat sweet potato once a week – and only about a quarter of one.

rice

Brown and wild rices are higher in fibre than white rice. I would have no more than a half-cup of rice (cooked) per week. Swap to quinoa or chia, as they are higher in protein.

pasta

No pasta – I tend to eat this to excess, unfortunately.

It's all about the quality of the carbohydrate that you are eating.

bern's simple high protein bread recipe (gf)

2 eggs
1tsp salt
1 zucchini, grated
1 large carrot, grated
1tsp bicarb of soda
2 cups chickpea (besan) flour
½ cup organic coconut oil, melted
1tsp turmeric
2tbsp dukkah (Egyptian spice blend)

If the mixture feels a bit dry add in some yoghurt or hummus – a couple of tablespoons.

Pre-heat oven to 180°C degrees, fan forced. Mix all the ingredients together until just combined and pour into a loaf tin. Bake for about 50 minutes.

When cooked, it should look mid brown and probably cracked on top – when you insert a skewer it should come out clean.

You can substitute the spices for different versions – I've put in oregano, garlic, rosemary...

It lasts me a week and I eat it toasted. Enjoy!

rule #7

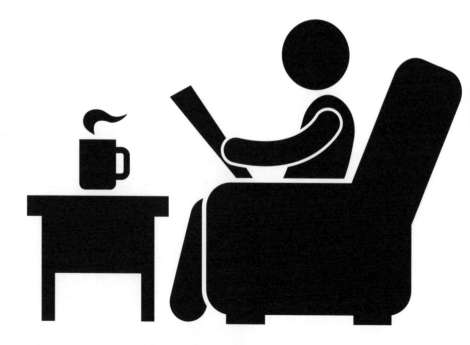

...i finish eating at 7pm and don't eat again until 10am...

overnight fasting is associated with increased cellular repair and fat burning, and it's a great opportunity to give your body a rest. who knew? it's amazing.

it's called
intermittent fasting
and it's not a diet,
but a pattern of
eating.

i fast for 15 hours
overnight, which
suits me.

why?

We live in an eating society. We're always eating and we don't tend to give ourselves a reasonable break from it. But we should, our bodies need it.

Overnight is an easy time to do an intermittent fast. Fasting lowers insulin levels and increases growth hormone levels, encouraging the breakdown of body fat and facilitating its use for energy.

As long as you don't compensate by eating more during the day, fasting can help you lower your overall daily calorie intake.

It's not hard to do – you're mostly sleeping anyway. I do this every night – except when my social life collides with it. That's when I cut myself some slack and start again the next day.

You may think that you'll wake up ravenous and run screaming to the fridge – but in actual fact that doesn't happen. It's almost the opposite. Weird, hey?

How I do it: breakfast after 10am, lunch around 2pm and dinner around 6pm. Because there are fewer hours between meals, I tend to eat less in-between. On a hungry day I might snack – nuts, cheese, veggies or a homemade sugar-free treat.

During my fasting period – 7pm to 10am – I drink green tea at night and strong coffee in the morning.

I find giving my body this rest period extremely beneficial as I feel so much better for it. I don't see myself stopping it, in either the short or long term. I love it.

rule #8

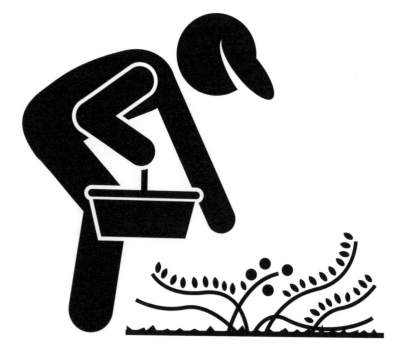

...i limit my fruit to one or two pieces a day. i eat the whole fruit – don't juice it...

berries will always
be my first choice.

also, i do not eat
dried fruits.

why?

don't juice it, or peel it, as you will lose the fibre, which is the good bit.

Fruit contains fructose – but not all fruits are equal. For example, berries, pineapples and kiwifruit have less fructose (sugar) than mangoes or pears. Choose well – but don't beat yourself up about it. Grapes are high in fructose, so I tend to stay away from those.

Eat the whole fruit, including the skin if possible. Don't juice it, otherwise you're losing all the good bits, namely the fibre, which helps you lose weight and aids in digestion. I limit the amount of fruit I eat because I want the fastest possible weight loss and fruit contains a lot of fructose/sugar – **and I am on a mission.**

Sometimes, I will only have one serving a day, usually berries, which are lower in fructose and high in fibre. Though perhaps I'm scarred from when I was a kid and would come home from school and say, 'I'm starved.' My mum would always say, 'Have a piece of fruit.' Aaaaahhh!

Eat fruits when they're in season – they are generally fresher. A farmers' market is a good place to buy fresh fruit and veg – really fresh and natural.

Dried fruits are generally high in fructose/ sugars. In some cases, they contain as much sugar as lollies (candy). A half-cup serving of dates contains about 55g of fructose per serving, which is the equivalent of 14 teaspoons of sugar. Regardless of where it has come from, your body treats these sugars the same way – turning it into fat – so I avoid dried fruits.

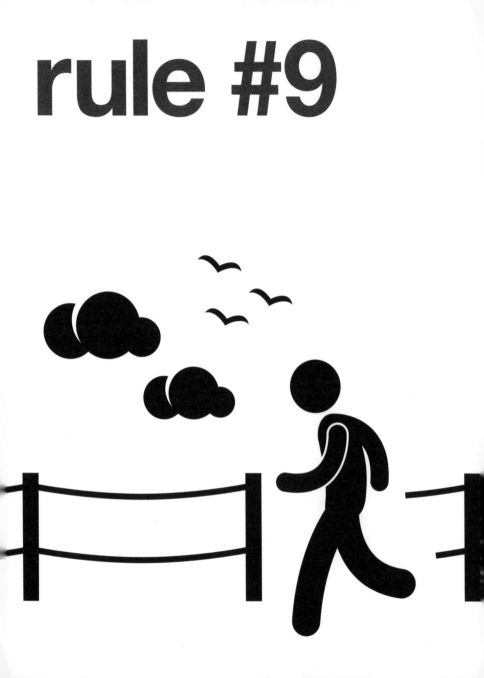

…i walk at least 10,000 steps a day or exercise for the equivalent…

wear a pedometer or download a walking app – it's easier than you think, and i think of it as 'my time'. go for a walk and listen to music or a podcast. i also come back in a better mood.

this is an important rule: exercise is great for my mental wellbeing and feeling good helps me stay on track.

10,000 steps a day is a rough equivalent to the guideline to do 150 minutes of activity a week – i.e. 25 minutes every day. Everyone from the US Surgeon General to the UK NHS to Australia's Department of Health recommends this. It's enough to reduce your risk of disease and help you lead a longer, healthier life. The benefits are many: lower BMI, reduced waist size, increased energy, and less risk of developing Type II diabetes and heart disease.

On average, a chocolate bar is 270 calories – to burn that off, you'd have to walk for an hour. If you want to actually lose weight but not change your eating habits, you'll need to exercise practically full-time.

why?

exercise burns fat, makes you feel fabulous and helps in general wellbeing. also it increases your muscle mass, which helps burn fat faster.

I don't know about you, but I absolutely do not have time to turn into a gym bunny.

Samuel Klein, MD at Washington University's School of Medicine, says: 'Decreasing food intake is much more effective than increasing physical activity to achieve weight loss.' No kidding!

Luckily for me and, hopefully, you, serious weight loss is mostly about the food – combined with a reasonable amount of exercise. Ditch the Lycra, get out your trackie, and start walking.

When you do get the desire to do more – and you will, believe it or not! – I suggest doing

weights as well as cardio such as walking, running, etc. Weight-training builds muscle – which not only makes you look more toned and slimmer, but muscle also burns fat. Win-win!

And, yes – exercise does make you hungrier, so don't pig out after it. Have a healthy snack and plenty of water instead. You'll feel doubly as good!

Exercise alone will never be enough to lose a significant amount of weight, because you have to do a TON in order to burn large amounts of fat. **That's why it is so important what you put in your mouth.**

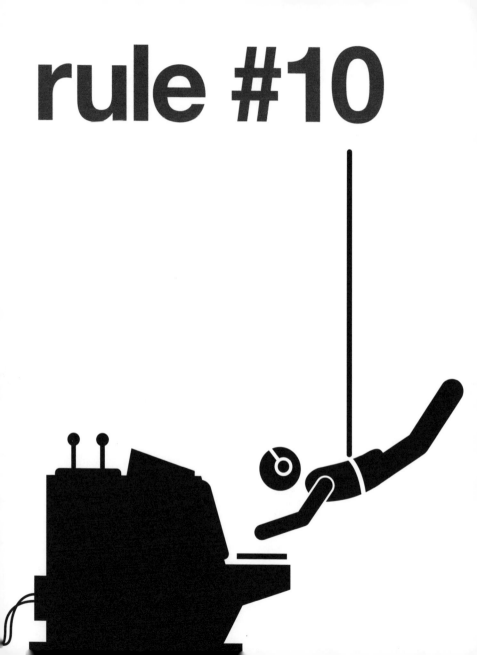

...i always read food labels...

why?

you need to know the ingredients in what you are buying and eating.

knowledge will speed up your weight loss.

let's face it, food labels are confusing... however, there's an easy rule – the shorter the label, the better. when there are lots of ingredients, it usually means more processing.

For example, canned chickpeas. The ingredient list: chickpeas and water. Great!

Generally, the fewer ingredients, the better. Stay away from anything with trans fats, as well as significant added sugar and salt. Remember, 4g is a teaspoon.

When I first started reading labels, if I saw an ingredient I didn't recognise, I wouldn't buy it. As a rule, ingredients are listed by order of volume – i.e. the first ingredient listed comprises the majority of the product.

Think about this: you don't need a food label on an apple. The best food for you is a whole ingredient. Really, anything that requires a food label – or has a TV ad – is a bit suspect, and the smaller the number of ingredients the better. But in reality… we're all busy and sometimes convenience wins out.

Just be smart about what you throw in the trolley and what you are going to feed your family – especially your kids. Teach them how to eat properly. It will save them from having the weight issues that you have had.

I ask my daughter to run on ahead of me and find the can of tomatoes with the lowest sugar amount. It's great – she's learning, plus saving me time. Win-win.

Doing this will quickly become a habit. You know those lean and healthy people standing in the supermarket aisles studying labels? That will soon be you!

rule #11

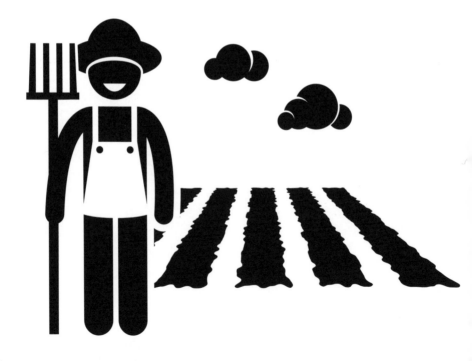

...i eat
whole
or clean
foods...

such as: eggs,
vegetables, fish,
meat, fruit (the
whole fruit),
grains, beans,
dairy, nuts.

fresh or whole
foods are single-
ingredient foods,
usually with no
ingredient list. they
can be combined
with other single
ingredients to
make delicious
meals.

why?

it's back to simplicity.
shop simply.

You know exactly what you're getting – there are no hidden sugars or fats or synthetic chemicals.

There is a *reason* why most slim celebrities that I work with have specific dietary requirements – it's because *they are all eating clean*, not because they are being difficult..

I also try to eat fruit and veggies only when they're in season – why eat six-month-old canned fruit or something that's been stored or treated with gas to preserve it?

When I was working on an ad for a supermarket chain, I went out to a storage dungeon for apples and it wasn't pretty – more like pretty gross. Stick to fresh and organic if you can.

I prefer organic chicken, grass-fed beef, free-range pork... Buy meats and fish where the animals are treated as humanely as possible.

Adding spices and seasoning to your food boosts flavour and taste, which will help you feel satisfied. In winter, I use my slow cooker and in summer, I make lots of salads – simple!

rule #12

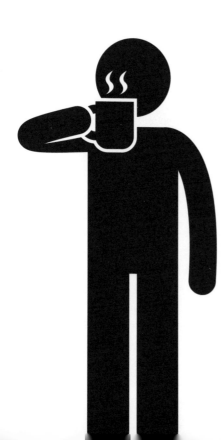

...i drink coffee first thing...

why?

i do this first thing in the morning when i wake up, then wait to have my breakfast at 10am.

The caffeine kick-starts my metabolism. It's a tip from some of the celebrity fitness gurus and athletes that I've worked with. They all say the same thing about the morning coffee – plus, it helps keep me regular… bonus!

The caffeine in coffee increases the rate at which your body burns calories. I stick to two coffees per day. I drink mine with a touch of milk (it's called a piccolo) – full-fat, of course. The reason I only want a touch of milk is that it is lower in calories than, say, a full latte; which contains a full cup of milk and, therefore, triple the calories.

If you have issues with caffeine such as headaches or jitters, avoid it, and definitely don't give it to children.

rule #13

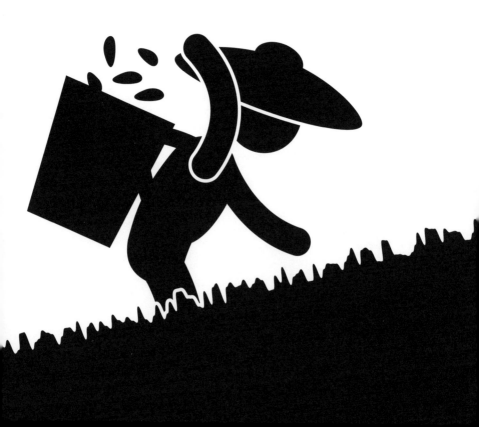

...i drink green tea over any other tea... why?

the active ingredient in green tea, EGCG – a naturally occurring and potent antioxidant – increases the rate at which fat is burned in your body.

Green tea, which is one of the least processed teas, has many other benefits including lowering cholesterol, but this antioxidant is key to weight loss.

Look for brands that contain sensha (ground green tea leaves), this means higher levels of the antioxidant EGCG. Most tea packaging has the level of antioxidant written on the box. I look for the highest levels when I am purchasing tea.

One to two cups of green tea have been proven to be beneficial to health. I like the taste, but 10 cups is my upper limit.

Remember, green tea contains caffeine and, as with coffee, don't drink it if you suffer side-effects. And don't serve green tea to children.

rule #14

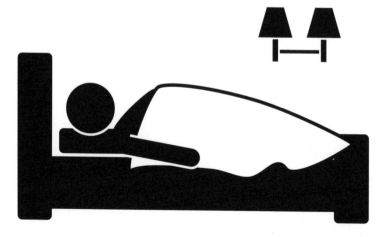

...i get nine hours of sleep a night...

sleep has been
shown to improve
your mental
wellbeing, while
poor sleep is
associated with
obesity and
weight gain.

i like eight to nine
hours per night,
but try to aim for
seven and a half
hours – at the
very least.

why?

we all need sleep
– it's a no-brainer!

Eating and sleeping are two basic human functions and they are closely intertwined – there are foods that are associated with improved sleep, such as leafy greens, and there are others that are associated with poorer sleep quality, such as fatty fast foods.

When I'm super-tired, I make poor decisions for my weight... **like reaching for cookies or hunting through my daughter's bedroom to find the remnants of her party sweets – desperate, really.**

It's self-sabotaging behaviour and I'm better off not exposing myself to it if I can help it. If I'm well-rested, my brain is sharper and I have the willpower to keep going. When I first started my Big Weightloss, I went to bed early, for two reasons. One, to stay away from food and break the bad habit of late-night eating,

accumulated over many years. Two, my research showed me the serious benefits of a good night's sleep. It helped that my nine-year-old liked that I was in bed early too.

Personally, I like to sleep more in winter and find I require less sleep in summer. Our circadian rhythms can make us feel that way – so if you're sleeping more or less at different times of the year, don't worry about it. It's Mother Nature.

Sometimes, getting plenty of sleep simply isn't possible... I get that. Just do your best.

According to a study of men by scientists at Sweden's Uppsala University, they burned up to 20% less energy the day after one night of sleep deprivation. Yikes!

rule #15

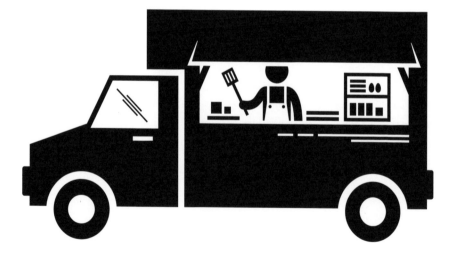

...I don't eat fast foods (usually)... why?

Fast foods are cheap, convenient and, let's face it, can be damn tasty – when I'm actually eating them. But usually, after I've finished devouring them, I don't feel so great.

Unfortunately, fast food is mostly filled with sugar, bad fats and salt – not good for you. That's why you feel so terrible after you've eaten them, not to mention the guilt. Luckily, there are some exceptions... Phew!

Such as:
Japanese – sushi, brown nori rolls
Vietnamese – low-carb rice paper rolls, pho
Lebanese – chicken or lamb and salad
Mexican – beans and salad and fish

Hunt around. There are plenty of good options once you know what to look for – think fresh, whole foods that are not deep fried.

you've gotta live in the real world! it's not possible to eat perfectly at every meal – sometimes, you just need to eat something, quick.

but try to make smart choices when you're choosing what to put in your precious body. you're in control.

rule #16

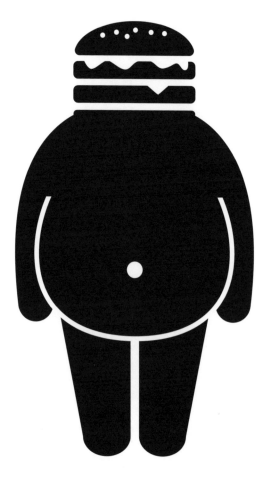

...i keep to a 'normal' portion size...

food portion sizes have gone up and up over the past few decades.

before you go
back for more,
give yourself 20
minutes to digest
what you've eaten
and decide if
you're still hungry.

in other words,
wait. take a
breather – *you're
not going to
starve in the next
20 minutes.*

why?

The movie *Supersize Me* is a good example of out-of-control portions, particularly in fast foods. Not to mention the show *Man vs Food*, which celebrates the enormous portion sizes that have become almost commonplace in the US, Australia and the UK.

It's easy to control your portion size at home – but when eating out, it's tempting to consume everything you've been served... even after you've had enough. *Stop when you feel satisfied, not full*.

Remember – a piece of meat or fish should be *the size of your palm*, and the rest of the plate should be lots of veggies or salad.

Follow it up with a home-made, sugar-free dessert if you like.

It takes 20 minutes for the brain to get the signal from your stomach that you're full – that's a medical fact!

Try using a smaller plate – it will look like you've got a bigger meal. Plates have increased in size over the years and the temptation is to fill the whole plate. Sounds dumb, but it actually works. And wait till you're actually hungry to eat – simple but effective.

rule #17

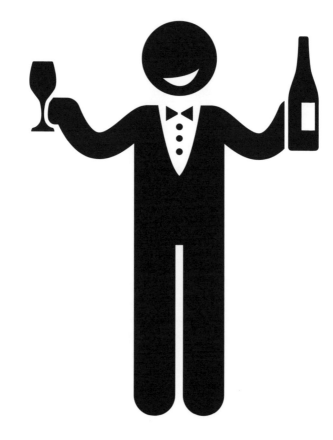

...i limit my alcohol...

why?

i'm not a big drinker, but occasionally i like to have a drink and extra occasionally, i like to really have a drink – if you know what i mean...

I've ditched high-sugar alcoholic drinks as the sugar will be stored as body fat if not used as energy. Instead, I drink a vodka-lime soda – real limes, not cordial, and fizzy water. Possibly on a night of dancing, I could get away with a bit more, as I would be burning up more energy.

I generally don't consume alcohol during the week. On the weekends, I may have one drink – but mostly it's easier to have none, as one can turn into three, which turns into six... And I'm more likely to eat unhealthy food if I'm drinking alcohol, so I try to avoid it.

And without alcohol, I wake up feeling fresher. This gets more and more true as I get older.

Admittedly, when I'm on holiday I loosen this rule... just a bit... What's a Bali sunset without a mojito with my friends? But try to avoid bad habits such as sinking a bottle of wine a night.

Alcohol interferes with the way fat metabolises – one more reason to limit it.

rule #18

...i eat my leafy greens with a good fat... why?

eat your (large quantity of) leafy greens (seriously, go crazy on leafy greens) with a good fat such as avocado or a good quality extra-virgin olive oil. this helps you absorb the vitamins.
it's also tastier.

some examples of leafy greens are

Rocket (arugula)

Kale

Lettuce

Spinach

Basically, if it's green and it's leafy get it on your plate!

some examples of good natural fats are

Avocados

Salmon and oily fishes – sardines, etc

Nuts including natural peanut butter

Sunflower, sesame and pumpkin seeds

Olives

Extra-virgin olive oil

Cheese (in moderation)

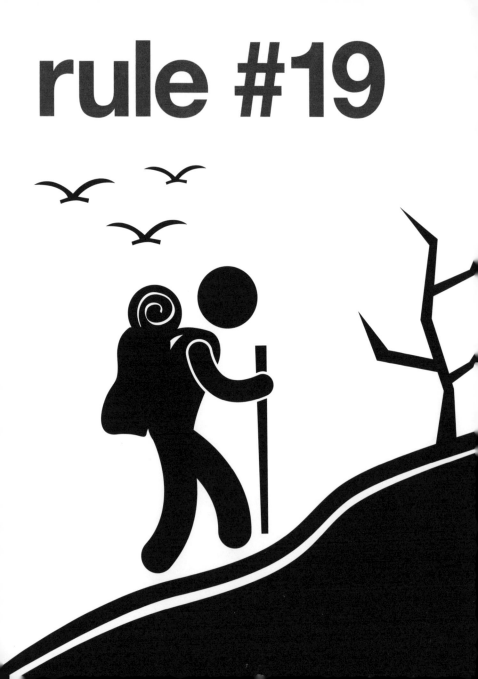

...i always carry snacks...

when i'm out
or working on
location, i take
snacks with me
– i don't want to
get caught out
hungry with little
to choose from.

which?

snack suggestions

Raw unprocessed nuts

Cut-up veggies

Berries

Hummus

Boiled eggs

Cheese

80% or 90% dark chocolate

Homemade smoothie: fresh fruit, veggies, ice/water

Sugar-free snacks – there are heaps of recipes online

Raw unprocessed nuts – a healthy daily intake is 30g or approximately ONE of the following serving sizes:

- 20 almonds
- 15 cashews
- 20 hazelnuts
- 15 macadamias
- 15 pecans
- 2 tablespoons of pine nuts
- 30 pistachio kernels
- 9 walnut kernels

A zip-lock bag is my best friend, especially on fashion and advertising shoots. You should see the food that's offered: chocolate, lollies, pastries… If I'm not prepared with my yummy snacks, then possible disaster.

rule #20

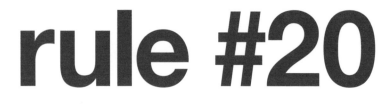

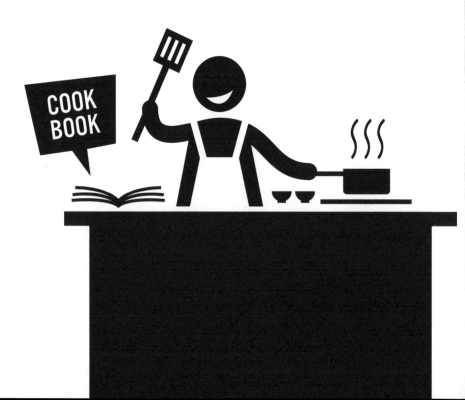

...prepare for your day/week...

'if you fail to prepare, then prepare to fail.'

– benjamin franklin

why?

snacks

When you're out or at work and won't be able to access good food choices, bring snacks and lunch with you. I start eating at 10am every day, so I bring boiled eggs, nuts and two slices of my Simple High Protein Bread with me.

shopping

It's easier to be healthy when you have all the right stuff in your cupboards and fridge. Keep your kitchen well-stocked and junk-free to make it easier to prepare meals for the whole family.

special occasions

When I'm going somewhere and I know there will be tempting foods, I try to eat beforehand. The hungrier I am, the less in control I am, if I'm being honest. So I prevent that.

sweet

When I'm feeling in control, I will occasionally allow myself a small bit of something sweet. This can get out of control quickly, so I have to judge my mood and be honest with myself about how in control I really am... it's usually less than I think, in all honesty. Remember these two words: *special occasion.* This is not an everyday activity!

sometimes

Occasionally I double the amount of a meal I'm cooking and freeze half for another time – this is handy for times when I'm busy.

supermarkets

Don't go shopping hungry! It's a recipe for disaster.

rules for the mind

sometimes i think
that successful
weight loss really
all starts in the mind.

rule #21

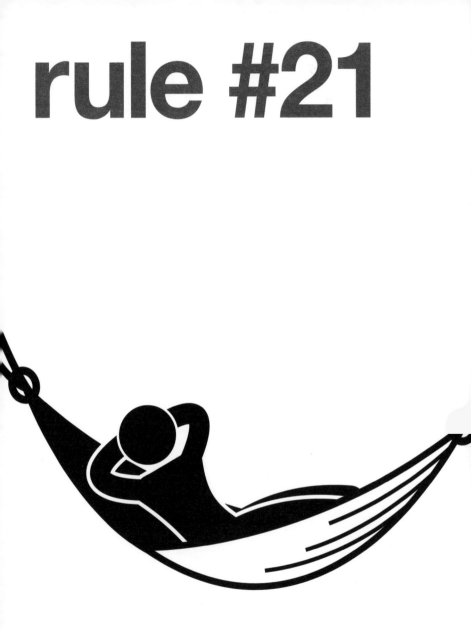

...i listen to my body...

why?

stop eating when you feel like you've had enough. remember, it takes 20 minutes for your brain to get the signal that you're full.

When you eat, focus on how your stomach feels through the entire meal. This is probably something that you will need to retrain yourself for, as you have probably been overeating for a while.

I had been overeating for, ooh, about 20 years... I remember I had to make a conscious effort to do this for the first couple of weeks of my Big Weightloss.

As you become full, the empty feeling in your stomach will be replaced with a gentle pressure. As soon as you feel this, stop eating; if the fullness is uncomfortable, you overate.

And if you feel like throwing up or lying down you really, really overate... It's about listening to your body.

rule #22

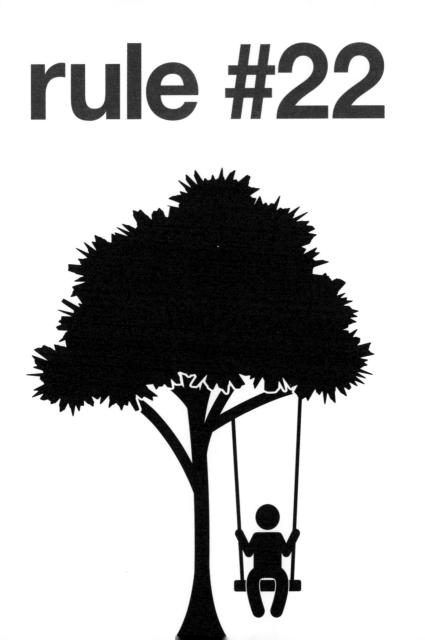

...I try my best not to get stressed...

stress can be linked to weight gain.

why?

it's all got to do with cortisol, a hormone released by your body in times of stress.

Cortisol can be associated with fat storage in the body. And some people notice an increase in appetite when they're stressed. Nooooooooo!

This one's different for everybody, but for me, it's a definite weight-gainer. When I was under considerable stress for a few years, I developed this truck tyre around my upper stomach area.

Could it be that the stress made me want to eat more comfort foods? This was definitely true. But it could also have been down to the link between cortisol and increased abdominal fat.

Try to have fun and look at the lighter side of life. I also try to appreciate the little things like the smells of spring, beautiful flowers etc. I try to notice the good around me and take time out once in a while.

So don't stress the small stuff, it's not worth it.

rule #23

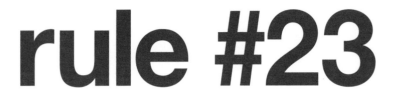

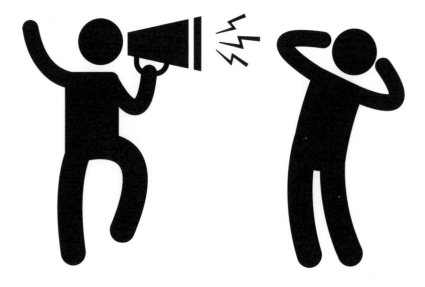

...i don't believe conventional wisdom about weight loss...

we can't believe
what we're told
about how to
lose weight when
there's an obesity
epidemic.

why?

make your own truth.

Conventional wisdom means those old sayings that you've heard a million times, like:

They're overweight, they must be lazy
They don't have the willpower to lose weight
Exercise more and eat less and you'll lose weight
Just exercise more
Don't eat junk food
Eat low-fat
Eat low-calorie or count calories
Eat six meals a day
It's your fault you're fat

These sayings are all flawed and some are flat-out lies.

My personal favourite is 'just eat low-fat' – that is crap! Most 'low-fat' foods have been filled with sugar and other nasties. Why on earth would you want to eat those? Unfortunately, we all bought into the 'low-fat' diet phase.

Most of us consumed low-fat food believing it must be better for us – this has turned out to be untrue. Just look around you!

rule #24

...hunger is not your friend...

it's not?

when you increase
your intake of healthy
fats and fibre, you
may notice you feel
fuller for longer.

forget the old belief
that if you're feeling
hungry, you are
somehow being
a good dieter.

it's not true.

It's emotionally taxing to fight hunger cravings and you usually end up losing anyhow... then feel depressed... We've all been on that downwards spiral.

Don't let yourself get too hungry or desperate for food. If you feel shaky, you've probably gone too long without eating – which ends up leading to poor decision-making.

When you eat well, you should feel satisfied for about four hours. If you do happen to get hungry, have a snack – simple. Make sure you carry healthy nibbles with you at all times, just in case.

Know your weak times. For me, it's around 4pm and sometimes, just after dinner. I make sure I'm prepared with 90% dark chocolate or some nuts.

It's harder to stick to a healthy and balanced diet when you're starving. It's much easier if you listen to your body and eat when you feel a bit hungry.

Give yourself every chance to succeed and you will!

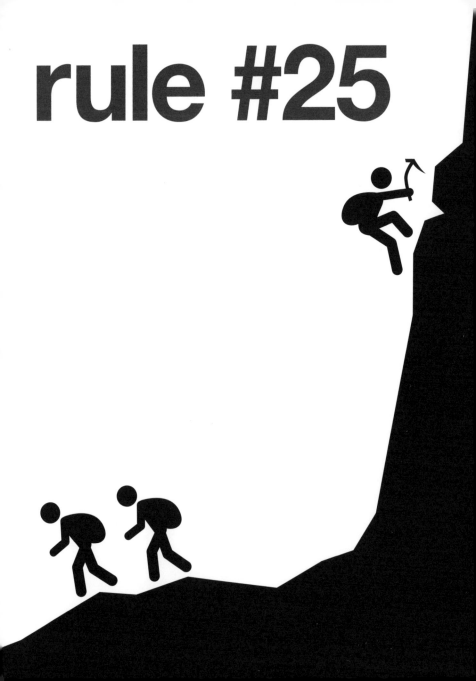

rule #25

...i handle my sweet tooth cravings...

how?

once i stopped
consuming
truckloads of
sugar, my taste
buds adapted.
now, i can taste
the real sweetness
in foods – even
vegetables.
isn't that amazing?

i no longer want extra-sweet foods, as i find them sickly. before i started the big weightloss, i was cynical of this claim – but it's true.

If you have a sweet tooth, then own it and be prepared. It's a good idea to make yourself a sugar-free treat – there are lots of recipes online. I always have something like this in the fridge, sometimes made with fructose-free rice malt syrup. Other than these snacks, don't torment yourself by keeping sugary stuff in the house – if it's available, it's easier to give in to temptation. Don't do that to yourself.

I recently went to a concert and my partner bought me some normal chocolate to 'celebrate' (I know, WTF?). After eating a considerable amount (double WTF!) I nearly vomited. I felt really sick, really quickly. Lesson learned: I was NOT missing sugar. After that, it became even easier to say no to sweets and candy.

Look for dark chocolate with 80 or 90% cacao content. 85% dark chocolate contains minimal sugar (2.5g, or just over half a teaspoon per 20g serving) and because it has a strong taste, it's hard to pig out on.

Dark chocolate also has a host of health benefits (when eaten in moderation):

Cocoa beans contain flavanols, which have antioxidant effects that reduce the cell damage connected to heart disease, help lower blood pressure and improve vascular function.

There are more flavanols and less sugar in dark chocolate than milk chocolate. I eat two pieces a day, as a treat.

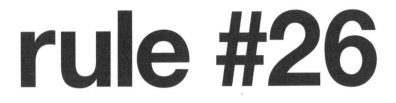

rule #26

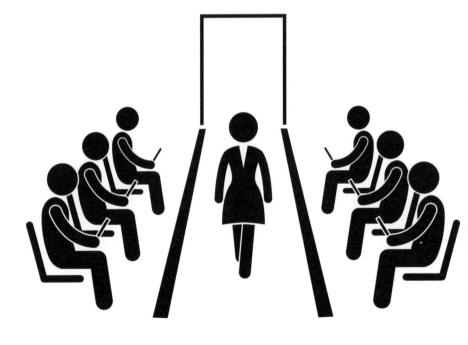

...take the media with a grain of salt (not literally)...

hmmm?

**it's hard to be fat
– in fact, it really
SUCKS.**

how can you lose weight when supposedly healthy food is full of stuff that makes you fat? it's impossible.

As well as being unhealthy, there are so many social issues that go with being overweight. Most importantly, the majority of overweight people I know don't like their bodies at all and will constantly put themselves down. Women are experts at this.

It is so frustrating to lose weight and regain it, again and again. Then we blame ourselves for our failure. But by now you should know it's mostly not your fault – and I'm pretty pissed at food companies. Cut yourself some slack – it's not all your doing.

There is such pressure, especially for young girls, to be beautiful and super-slim like models in magazines. And I'm one of the people perpetuating that myth, as I do the hair and makeup that makes those models look the way they do. Before the picture is even taken, they usually spend at least one and a half hours in hair and makeup. Then the picture is Photoshopped for 'flaws'. What you see is absolutely not reality.

I remember working on an ad for a mainstream diet product overseas and the model was gorgeous – tall, size 8 (US 4-6). The pictures were Photoshopped within an inch of her life because they thought her bum and legs looked too big – mental! But it happens all the time.

But, to be perfectly honest, I'm not aiming for skinny, either. It's not attractive to me. I much prefer the look of the models who are a healthy size 12-14 (US 10-12) with boobs and a bum – that's what I aspire to. Fit and curvy, please, like Australian model Laura Wells – who also does great work with the environment.

What I'm trying to say is, don't aspire to unachievable media perfection – it's not real. Be the best that you can be – it's enough. In fact, it's more than enough.

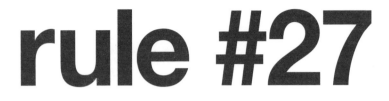

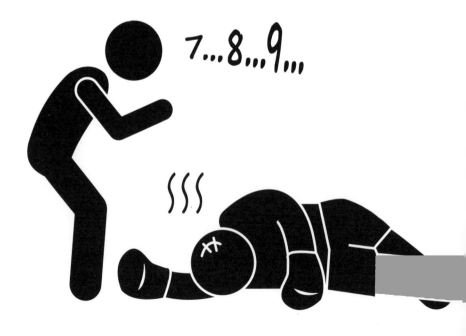

...stop counting calories...

really?

it's annoying, time-consuming, and you don't need to when you eat according to my rules.

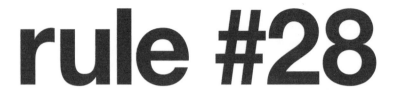

rule #28

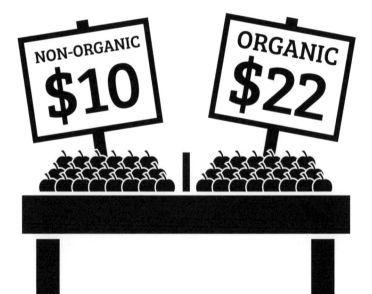

NON-ORGANIC
$10

ORGANIC
$22

...organic is not necessarily good...

really?

organic whole foods are excellent – but processed organic foods are not.

You need to check the labels to make sure what you're eating is not high in hidden fats, sugars or chemicals.

And sometimes, the identical food is in the 'normal' aisles at half the price – when ingredients are shelved in the health food area and stamped as organic, they suddenly cost a bomb.

Some supposed health foods are really candy bars in disguise, with massive sugar content. Don't assume that the organic and health food aisle in the supermarket is all good – remember, read your food labels.

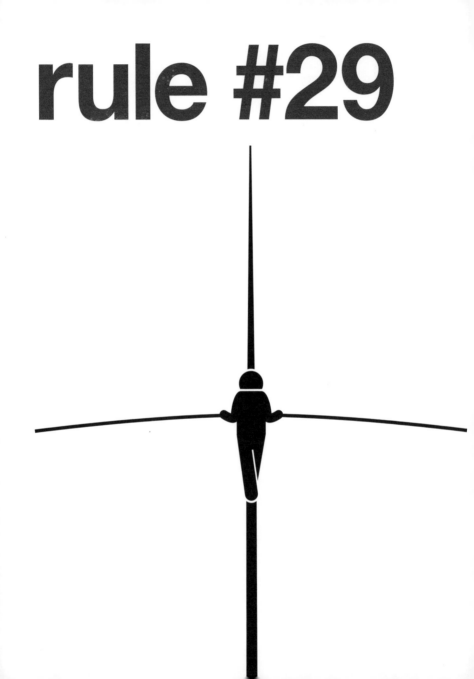

...i use substitutes for sugar... which?

I don't like artificial sweeteners – I find them too processed and the taste unpleasant. Here are some of them – even the names of them sounds unnatural, no wonder I don't like them.

- Saccharin
- Aspartame
- Acesulfame-K
- Sucralose
- Neotame

Plus, the jury is still out on whether artificial sweeteners are OK or harmful to your body in the long term. Why risk it?

The most 'natural' artificial sweetener is stevia, which is a calorie-free plant extract about 200 times as sweet as table sugar when refined – a little goes a long way. But I'm not keen on its aftertaste.

my favourite sugar substitute is rice malt syrup. i do use it sparingly as it still has a high glycaemic index and nutritionally it has few benefits other than being tasty, but it is fructose-free.

rule #30

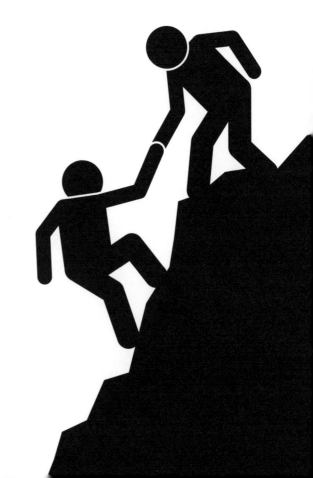

...be kind
to yourself
and think
positively...

ok, then?

remember, if you
slip up: tomorrow
is another day, and
another chance
to be healthy. in
other words, be
kind to yourself
and *make yourself
a priority.*

Go for that walk or take the kids on their scooters, just keep moving – it will help with your state of mind and make it easier to stay on track. Remember that *success is just outside of your comfort zone* – a total cliché but also totally true.

Sometimes, I think that staying on track is more mental than anything else. If I'm angry or feeling flat or tired, it's easier to eat foods that are not good for me. **Yes, I'm a bit of an emotional eater.**

I believe that long-term weight loss is about changing your internal messages to yourself. Say to yourself: you can do it, you're going well, good on you. Be your own best friend and coach – positive reinforcement will help you in the short- and long-term. *Positive actions lead to positive results.* Try to make this a daily habit.

I also find talking to other people about their healthy habits and sharing some of mine is inspiring – if you can find other people who are on the same healthy journey as you, even better. If you can surround yourself with positive people intent on positive change that is fantastic. Talking helps – *we're all in this together!*

Visualise yourself living the life you want. *Believe you can do it – because you can.* Another totally true cliché!

rule #31

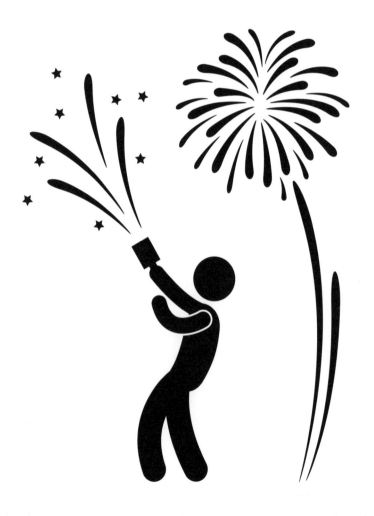

...celebrate
your success
and tolerate
your plateaus...

why?

i reward myself with
a movie, clothes
or earrings...
anything but sugary
processed food. it's
almost enough of
a reward to see the
scales go down
and down.

'people wait until they reach their goal weight before they think they're allowed to feel good about themselves... and that's just dumb!'

– claryssa humennyj-jameson

It's about being good to yourself... being your own biggest champion. Do it because it's important – just like you are. I positively love shopping for clothes now. And I don't seem to be as invisible to shop assistants, for some reason... Funny, that!

While I'm transitioning sizes, I buy my clothes at op shops (charity shops/thrift stores) or markets – I don't want to spend heaps on brand-new stuff I'm going to shrink out of. I also like eBay for this.

If your weight plateaus – i.e., you don't lose anything for a week... or three – don't worry. It's part of the journey of weight loss and happens to

everyone. I plateaued for more than three weeks and, yes, it drove me crazy... but it did pass.

And after a weekend away hiking in Tasmania, I actually gained weight – 1.5kg (3lb)! Initially, I was super-disappointed as I had exercised and eaten well. But as my clothes were looser and I didn't feel like I'd gained anything, I put it down to increased muscle (which weighs more than fat).

Sometimes, the scales are wrong. Before you begin your Big Weightloss journey, take your measurements and weight and put them in the About You section at the back of this book. Your shrinking measurements are another great way to see your progress.

how
to get
started

...take on one thing at a time...

...and take it one day at a time...

how to get started.

Right before I first began this style of eating, I saw my doctor for blood tests and a check-up to see where I was at. After three months I saw her again and we were both astounded at the improvements I had made.

It's a good idea to see your doctor before you start any weight-loss plan – in case there is a medical issue you might not be aware of.

Next, you'll need to do a big healthy shop at the supermarket.

And you have to clean out your kitchen cupboards of all the unhealthy foods. Give them away, donate them, just get rid of them!

If they're in the house, within arm's reach, it's far easier to give into temptation.

Buy a pedometer or an app for your phone that counts steps. Devices that measure your sleep and steps are great. Get a good night's sleep, then get up and weigh and measure yourself – you're good to go with the first step.

Week by week, I took on one hard task and one easy task, until I was doing all these habits together. Obviously it's going to vary from person to person, depending on your habits and what you find hard and easy.

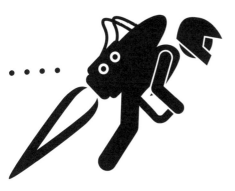

week 1

I started off by getting rid of processed foods and adding what I thought was an easy habit… walking.

week 2

I gave up sugar (a harder one for me) and added in good sleeping habits.

week 3

I cut back on my carbs and added another easy one… no soft drinks.

And so on. Introducing new things each week gives you the best chance of success. Some weeks are going to be easier than others – expect that, but persevere. The pay-off is weight loss – lots of it.

However you approach this, you're off and running to a healthier and slimmer you.

perseverance and persistence is key.

what's in my cupboards

dairy

Eggs – free range
Yoghurt – full-fat Greek
Milk – full-fat
Sour cream
Cheese – I love Persian feta and haloumi
Butter/ghee

vegetables

Cauliflower (good for cauliflower rice)
Avocado
Carrots
Red peppers – I roast these
Sweet potatoes
Zucchini – for spiralizing
Tomatoes – I like cherry ones
Pumpkin – love these roasted
Leafy greens
Mushrooms – yum on toast at brekkie
Whatever else you like – I don't tend to buy
corn or white potatoes

fruit

Berries
Apples
Oranges
Seasonal fruits

meat and fish

Minced pork – free range
Beef – grass-fed
Salmon – if I have the $!
Tuna – canned, ethically caught
Chicken – organic
Bacon – free-range

nuts and pulses

Nuts – buy a variety of raw and unsalted ones
Lentils – a variety of dried and canned
Beans – a variety of dried and canned
Pumpkin seeds – I use these in cooking bread

liquids

Coconut oil – raw and organic

Olive oil

Rice malt syrup – for my fructose-free desserts

Balsamic vinegar

Coconut – milk and cream

Apple cider vinegar with mother

store cupboard

Flours – lentil, chickpea, coconut

Chia seeds, quinoa

Rice – brown or wild

Oats – rolled ones, plain and unsweetened

Herbs and spices

Peanut butter – natural or organic (it's cheaper
in the main aisles than the health-food aisles)

Dark chocolate – with 80–90% cacao

Green tea bags

Coffee

Bottles of soda water

Small zip-lock bags

an example of a typical day, food-wise

drink water
first thing, with
all meals, and
throughout the
day, as well as
green tea.

7am – first thing

Coffee with a dash of full-fat milk (sometimes I have two)

10am – breakfast – this is when i first eat

One of the following:

• 2 pieces protein bread, ½ avocado, 2 slices bacon

• 1 piece protein bread, 2 poached eggs

• 30g bowl rolled oats with yoghurt and berries

• 1 tablespoon chia seeds with yoghurt and berries

• 2 pieces Bern's protein bread, grilled with cheese and tomato

• 2 eggs scrambled in butter, mushrooms, bacon, spinach

2pm – lunch – it's quite simply a mix of protein and leafy greens

One of the following:

• A large bowl of soup – homemade with veggies or beans

• A large green salad with salmon or chicken

• Any combo of leafy greens and protein

• Raw salmon sashimi – I love Japanese food

4pm – snack

One of the following:

• 30g nuts – raw and unsalted

• Berries – a small handful

6pm – dinner

One of the following:

• Grilled fish or meat with vegetables or salad

• Coconut milk Thai curry – made with fish, chicken or vegetables and served with cauliflower rice

• Indian curry – as above

• Leafy greens with onion, tomato, fresh parmesan, dressed with olive oil and balsamic

6.45pm – snack

2 pieces of 80% dark chocolate

No more eating after 7pm.

finally...

you don't
need luck,
this will
work

don't go back to your previous bad habits and bad eating. learn what feels good for your body and mind and stick to it, because you deserve it.

Lots of people lose weight on fad diets, only to regain it back within five years – and more. Look at *The Biggest Loser* statistics – many of the contestants have regained the weight they lost, because in the real world it's not possible to exercise for hours each day. Who has that much free time? No one! My life is generally messy and busy.

Weight loss needs to be achievable. It's a long-term lifestyle change. Don't be one of those statistics – you will need to consistently stay away from sugar and processed foods.

It's a fine balance – if I'm feeling the pull to eat sugary foods, I know I need to wipe anything sweet off the menu for a bit. It is seriously addictive for me. And I've come to accept I can't handle it.

Twice a week, I weigh myself in my bra and knickers so that I can keep an eye on my progress. If I can do this then so can you.

believe in yourself.

maintenance

Once you've hit your goal weight or size, you can think about adding back a little bit more fruit, or a few more carbs – or maybe don't do the intermittent fast every night… It's really up to you.

You're going to give your body more of the healthy and nutritious foods that it deserves – I believe you won't fall back into bad habits because you will have learnt what feels good for your body. And you're on a life-long path to health.

Find a balance in food and lifestyle that you can live with, for life. The best possible life. Good luck.

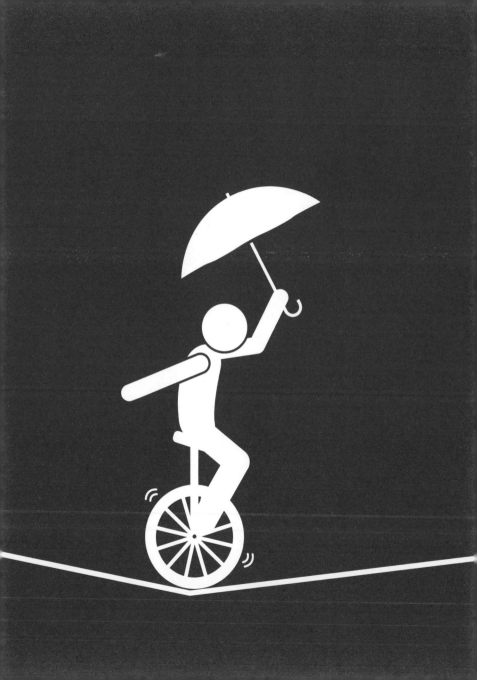

just some of the many medical studies i've read

Avena, Nicole M., Pedro Rada, and Bartley G. Hoebel. "Evidence for Sugar Addiction: Behavioral and Neurochemical Effects of Intermittent, Excessive Sugar Intake." Neuroscience and biobehavioral reviews 32.1 (2008): 20–39. PMC. Web. 21 July 2016.

DiNicolantonio JJ, Lucan SC The wrong white crystals: not salt but sugar as aetiological in hypertension and cardiometabolic disease Open Heart 2014;1:e000167. doi: 10.1136/openhrt-2014-000167

Mozaffarian D, Hao T, Rimm EB, Willett WC, Hu FB. Changes in diet and lifestyle and long-term weight gain in women and men. N Engl J Med. 2011;364:2392-404.

Jacobson M. Liquid Candy: How Soft Drinks are Harming Americans' Health. Washington, DC: Center for Science in the Public Interest; 2005.

2001 Feb 17;357(9255):505-8.

Relation between consumption of sugar-sweetened drinks and childhood obesity: a prospective, observational analysis. Ludwig DS1, Peterson KE, Gortmaker SL.

Institute of Medicine. Accelerating Progress in Obesity Prevention: Solving the Weight of the Nation. Washington, DC: National Academies Press; 2012.

Hung, H.C., et al., Fruit and vegetable intake and risk of major chronic disease. J Natl Cancer Inst, 2004. 96(21): p. 1577-84

The Visual Illusions of Food: Why Plates, Bowls, and Spoons Can Bias Consumption Volume
Brian Wansink1 and Koert van Ittersum2
1 AEM, Cornell, 110 Warren Hall, Cornell University, Ithaca, NY, 14850,
2 Marketing, Georgia Tech, 100 Dupree Hall, Atlanta, GA, 32196

Drinking water is associated with weight loss in overweight dieting women independent of diet and activity. Stookey JD, Constant F, Popkin BM. Obesity (Silver Spring, Md.), 2008, Sep.;16(11):1930-7381.

University Of Minnesota. "15-year Study Shows Strong Link Between Fast Food, Obesity And Insulin Resistance." ScienceDaily. ScienceDaily, 19 January 2005. <www.sciencedaily.com/releases/2005/01/050111152135.htm>.

A Systematic Review of the Literature on Intermittent Fasting for Weight Management
Catherine Hankey1, Dominika Klukowska1 and Michael Lean1
April 2015
The FASEB Journal

Association between reduced sleep and weight gain in women. Patel SR1, Malhotra A, White DP, Gottlieb DJ, Hu FB.
Author information
1Division of Pulmonary and Critical Care Medicine, University Hospitals of Cleveland, Case Western Reserve University, Cleveland, OH 44106, USA. srp20@case.edu

Acute sleep deprivation reduces energy expenditure in healthy men.
Benedict C1, Hallschmid M, Lassen A, Mahnke C, Schultes B, Schiöth HB, Born J, Lange T.
First published April 6, 2011, doi: 10.3945/ajcn.110.006460
Am J Clin Nutr June 2011
vol. 93 no. 6 1229-1236

Dietary fiber and weight regulation.
Howarth NC1, Saltzman E, Roberts SB.
Author information
Jean Mayer USDA Human Nutrition Research Center on Aging at Tufts University, Boston, MA 02111, USA.

Caffeine and coffee: their influence on metabolic rate and substrate utilization in normal weight and obese individuals.
Acheson KJ, Zahorska-Markiewicz B, Pittet P, Anantharaman K, Jéquier E
2008 Mar;87(3):778-84.

Green tea extract ingestion, fat oxidation, and glucose tolerance in healthy humans.
Venables MC1, Hulston CJ, Cox HR, Jeukendrup AE.
Author information
Human Performance Laboratory, School of Sport and Exercise Sciences, The University of Birmingham, Birmingham, United Kingdom.

thanks to

Terence Langendoen, Lilli Langendoen, Claire Fisers, Jakki and Johann Bilsborough, Myrtle Jeffs, Mel Krienke, Claryssa Humennyj-Jameson, Kylie Starling, Felicite Phillips, Michael Heath, Harriet Reuter Hapgood, Christian Lockwood, Jack Lockwood, Michael Lenihan, Julie Spalding, Lisa Tyler, Natalie Kirby plus all the models, art directors, clients, athletes, trainers and photographers that I have worked with that have talked to me about nutrition and have encouraged me – I thank you all.

follow bernadette online

@bigweightlossau

@littlebookbigweightloss

@littlebookofbigweightloss

pinterest.com/bernfish/the-little-book-of-big-weightloss/

thatdietbook.com

also available as an e-book